HOW NOT TO AGE COOKBOOK

HEALTHY RECIPES FOR LONGITIVITY INSPIRED BY DR GREGER'S TEACHINGS

Alice D. Ducker

COPYRIGHT

INTRODUCTION

Simmering on the stove is your fountain of youth; forget about wrinkle creams and miracle elixirs! Welcome to the "How Not to Age Cookbook," a colourful and tasty journey into the realm of long-term plant-based diet based on Dr. Michael Greger's ground-breaking research.

To be honest, I wasn't always an advocate for the kitchen. I too followed the illusive carrot of anti-aging, trailing through confusing mazes of fad diets and questionable supplements. However, discovering Dr. Greger's work was like a complete script change on ageing. His methodical approach, supported by an abundance of data, uncovered a straightforward truth: the most potent anti-aging weapon available to us is the food we consume.

This cookbook was created as a result. It's more than just a cookbook; it's a guide to rediscovering your health and energy via the colourful harmony of the plant life. Every page is bursting with the colours of vitality, from leafy greens that reduce inflammation to berries that are loaded with antioxidants. Along with innovative takes on comfort cuisine favourites like creamy pumpkin mac & cheese, you can sample Thai noodle bowls and Ethiopian lentil stews.

Yes, these recipes are based on science. But don't worry, making them won't need a lab coat. Every meal is painstakingly created to be a gastronomic explosion, a love letter to your taste senses that also contains elements that extend the life of food.

However, this book is a celebration of life rather than only physical nourishment. It's about eating meals that feed your soul as well as your body, while also sharing love and laughter. It's about reclaiming the delight of cooking, the enchantment of metamorphosis, and the ability of pleasure to reshape the story of ageing.

In his book "How Not to Age," Dr. Greger makes the case that becoming older need not equate to being ill. He focuses on methods supported by research to maximise lifespan and health, taking cues from "blue zones" where residents live very long lives. His main points are as follows:

Nutrition:

Plant-based whole foods: To achieve adequate nutrition and lower risk of chronic illnesses, give priority to fruits, vegetables, legumes, and whole grains. Few animal products and processed foods: Reduce your intake of red meat, sugar-filled beverages, and processed meals since they all cause inflammation and chronic disease.

Particular nutrients: Foods high in substances that support cell health and lifespan include apples, tempeh, and mushrooms.

Way of life:

Frequent exercise: For the sake of your muscles and cardiovascular health, try to get in most days of the week with moderate-intensity exercise.

Good sleep: Set aside 7-8 hours each night to have the best possible physical and mental health.

Stress management: To lower inflammation and enhance general health, learn good coping mechanisms for stress, such as meditation or time spent in nature.

Additional elements

Social connection: Having strong social ties promotes happiness and wellbeing, both of which have a beneficial effect on life expectancy.

Life's purpose: Having a feeling of direction and significance in one's existence helps improve motivation and general wellbeing.

Overall message: According to Dr. Greger, we can greatly extend our lives and enhance our health by embracing a plant-based diet, emphasizing smart lifestyle choices, and developing an optimistic mindset. This will allow us to age in a manner that is both healthier and more lively.

The Three Foundations Of Greger's Teachings

With an emphasis on natural foods and few processed or animal-derived substances, Dr. Greger advocates a plant-based diet. Prioritising these important categories is what he suggests:

Antioxidants, fibre, and vitamins are abundant in fruits and vegetables, whichvpromote general well-being and help prevent illness. Complex carbs and fibre included in whole grains provide you long-lasting energy.

Legumes: A great way to get fibre, protein, and other important elements. Rich in protein, minerals, and good fats are nuts and seeds.

Cookbook Consistency: These ideas are supported by the "How Not to Age Cookbook" in a number of ways:

Focus on plants: A wide variety of vibrant fruits, vegetables, legumes, and nutritious grains can be found in the dishes, most of which are vegan or vegetarian. Minimum amount of processed components With as little processed food, harmful fats, or refined sugar as possible, the focus is on whole, fresh foods.

Rich in antioxidants, fibre, vitamins, minerals, and other vital elements that Greger stresses, the dishes showcase products that are nutrient-dense. The book doesn't compromise on flavour, even with its health-conscious theme.

Taste buds will be enticed and your body will be nourished by the inventive and varied cuisine.

For instance:

Or picture yourself enjoying a rich, creamy, spicy Thai coconut curry with tofu and veggies that is exploding with flavour and nutrition, or a colourful Mediterranean chickpea salad bowl that is full of protein, fibre, and antioxidants. These hardly scratch the surface of the cookbook's filling yet healthful selections.

Move Past Recipes:

Greger's ideas are integrated into the culinary philosophy in this book, which goes beyond just providing recipes. Together with dietary recommendations based on certain health issues, it offers meal planning advice and explains the science behind the nutritious foods.

In General:

In addition to being a cookbook, "How Not to Age Cookbook" is a useful manual for incorporating Dr. Greger's ideas into your cooking endeavours. Greger's goal of maximum health via a plant-based diet is aligned with your ability to prepare tasty, nutrient-rich meals that promote your health and well-being.

Though Dr. Greger's study and cookbook provide insightful information, it's important to customise his concepts to your own requirements and tastes. For individualised nutritional recommendations, speak with a healthcare provider. Go ahead and peruse the "How Not to Age Cookbook," and let Dr. Greger's

guidance guide you as you set off on a delightful and healthful culinary adventure!

Boosting Longitivity and Well-being Through Plant-based Diet

Rich in fruits, vegetables, whole grains, legumes, and nuts, a plant-based diet has a wealth of advantages for extending life and improving mental and physical health. How to do it is as follows:

Increased Longevity: Lower risk of chronic diseases: Diets based mostly on plants are naturally abundant in fibre, antioxidants, and vital vitamins and minerals and low in cholesterol, salt, and saturated and trans fats. This results in a decreased risk of stroke, heart disease, type 2 diabetes, several malignancies, and even Alzheimer's disease—all of which are significant causes of premature mortality.

Better cellular health: Rich in antioxidants, plant foods fight oxidative stress, avsignificant cause of ageing and age-related illnesses. Additionally, they support cellular regeneration and proper DNA repair, which may slow down the ageing process.

Weight management: Diets rich in fibre, which keeps you feeling fuller for longer and supports good digestion, tend to be naturally lower in calories and fat. This may help you maintain a healthy weight, which is another important component of long life.

Advantages for Well-Being:

Enhanced energy: Plant-based diets are full of vital nutrients and complex carbs, which keep you feeling energised all day. This may help you feel less worn out and have more energy overall, making you feel livelier and more engaged.

Enhanced mood and cognitive performance: Research indicates that eating a plant-based diet might lessen anxiety and sadness, boost mood, and even improve cognitive function. The profusion of antioxidants, vitamins, and minerals that promote brain function and neurotransmitter synthesis is probably the cause of this.

Enhanced immunity: Plant-based diets are abundant in vitamins and minerals, particularly vitamin C, which is critical for a robust immune system. You can prevent illnesses and maintain your health more often by doing this.

Better digestion: The high fibre content of plant-based diets naturally encourages regular bowel motions and good gut flora. This may result in less bloating and constipation, better digestion, and improved gut health in general.

The Anti-Ageing Eight in Action

All people want to live long, healthy lives. Science has discovered a wealth of nutritional knowledge concealed in the vivid hues of fruits and vegetables, the common bean, and the aromatic symphony of spices—all while the spring of youth is still elusive. These are the **Anti-Aging Eight**, eight essential components sewn into the fabric of lifespan, not just delicious foods.

Leafy Greens: The Natural Powerhouses Full with nutrients that are essential for life, kale, spinach, and collard greens are verdant champions. Packed with fibre, folate, vitamins C and K, and an array of phytonutrients, they help maintain the health and vibrancy of your cells. Consider them to be the natural equivalent of personal trainers, shaping your body from the inside out.

Beans: The Lowly Giants of Eternity Don't undervalue the powerful bean! Not only do beans taste great on your plate, but they are also superfoods for longevity since they are full of fibre, protein, and many vitamins and minerals. They are the hidden heroes of general health—they help control blood sugar, prolong feelings of fullness, and support your gut microbiota.

Antioxidant Jewels Berries: Natural candies, these little bursts of sweetness are brimming with antioxidants that scavenge free radicals, the cellular misfits that hasten the ageing process. Berries are a delicious way to add anti-aging magic to your day, from strawberries and açai to blueberries and raspberries.

The Little Titans of Nutrition Nuts and Seeds: Rich in fibre, protein, healthy fats, and an abundance of vitamins and minerals, walnuts, almonds, flaxseeds, andchia seeds are little nutritional powerhouses. They not only support healthy brain function but also lower inflammation, maintain a healthy heart, and provide your body with long-lasting energy

Spices Fragrant Medicine Remedies: Spices like garlic, ginger, cinnamon, and turmeric are more than simply flavour enhancers; they are aromatic representatives of the plant life. They have a multitude of health-promoting qualities and are strong anti-inflammatory agents. Consider them to be the natural alchemists inside, converting your food into scrumptious health-boosting concoctions.

Whole Grains The Steady and Slow Victorians: Replace your refined grains with brown rice, quinoa, oats, and whole wheat bread, which are whole grains. These slow-burning, high-fiber, vitamin- and mineral-rich energy sources also maintain stable blood sugar levels and provide you long-lasting energy. In the fight againstage-related deterioration, they are the steadfast soldiers.

Nature's Detox PatrolCruciferous Vegetables: Brussels sprouts, kale, broccoli, cauliflower, and other cruciferous vegetables are not only tasty but also powerful detoxifiers. They contain a lot of sulforaphane, which is a substance that keeps your cells clean and helps neutralise dangerous poisons. Consider them to be nature's internal cleansing brushes, ensuring optimal bodily functions.

Water The Vital Elixir: Water is the unsung hero of longevity, despite its seeming simplicity. It maintains your cells happy and plump, lubricates your joints, and removes pollutants. Try eight glasses a day, and you'll see inside bodily transformation.

Remember, the Anti-Aging Eight represent a colourful tapestry of delectable possibilities rather than a strict set of rules. Accept their variety, try new flavours, and allow your meals turn into an ode to long life and good health. You are creating the fabric of your own unique life narrative with each mouthful of a leafy green, each crunchy bean, and each blast of sweetness from berries.

Put an end to fad diets and adopt the Anti-Aging Eight's knowledge instead. Make your meals become experiments, your kitchen into a lab, and your taste sensations into guides. As you discover the mysteries these common heroes are hiding.

BEANS

Beans A Superfood with Unmatched Nutrition and Tasty Variety:

The lowly bean family, which includes kidney, black, lentil, and chickpeas, is a nutritious powerhouse that should take centre stage in your diet. Tightly packed with protein, fibre, vitamins, and minerals, they're not only healthful but also very adaptable, turning into a myriad of delectable and fulfilling recipes. Explore the dietary advantages of beans and discover their culinary versatility via a variety of dishes as we delve into the world of beans.

Nutritional Highlight:

Protein Powerhouse: Beans are a great plant-based protein that is needed for tissue growth and repair, which is why vegetarians and vegans should eat them. Eighteen grammes of protein, or three ounces of chicken, may be found in one cup of cooked lentils! Beans are a great source of fibre that may help with digestion, support gut health, and help you feel fuller for longer. In addition, this dietary fibre aids in cholesterol and blood sugar regulation. Iron, folate, potassium, magnesium, and phosphorus are just a few of the vitamins and minerals that beans are a vitamin and mineral bonanza full of.These nutrients support bone health, muscular function, red blood cell creation,and energy generation.

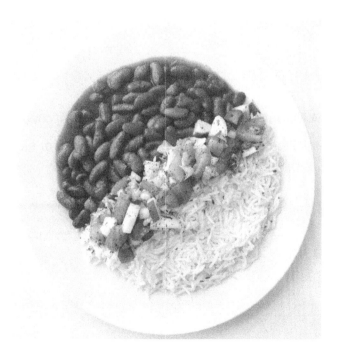

LENTIL LOVE

Lentil Soup with Roasted Vegetables: This hearty soup is packed with protein, fiber, and flavor. Roasting vegetables like carrots, onions, and peppers adds depth and sweetness

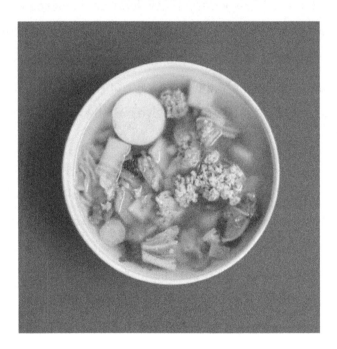

Moroccan Lentil Salad: A vibrant and refreshing salad with lentils, cucumbers, tomatoes, red onion, and a Moroccan-inspired dressing. Perfect for a light lunch or side dish.

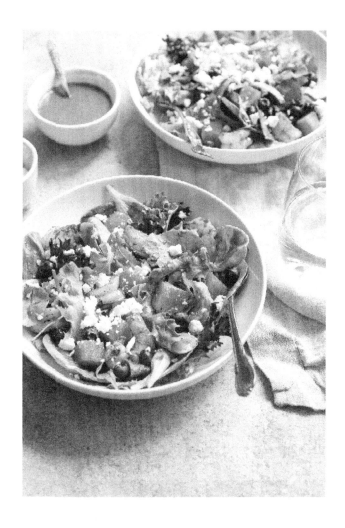

Indian Dal: A staple in Indian cuisine, dal is a lentil stew simmered with spices like turmeric, cumin, and coriander. Serve with rice or naan for a comforting and flavorful meal.

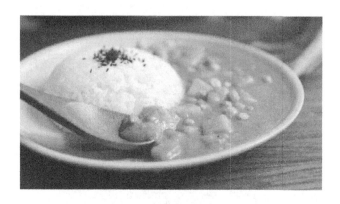

CHICKPEA CELEBRATION

Falafel: These crispy chickpea fritters are a Middle Eastern delight, perfect for pita bread sandwiches or served with hummus and vegetables.

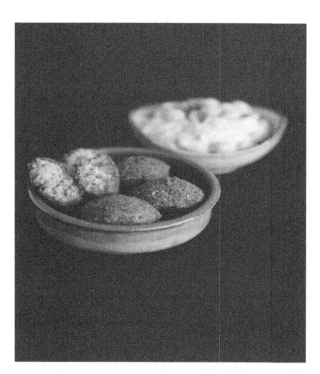

Indian chickpea dish with spices, onions, and tomatoes, known as chana masala. Serve this dish with roti or rice for a filling vegan supper.

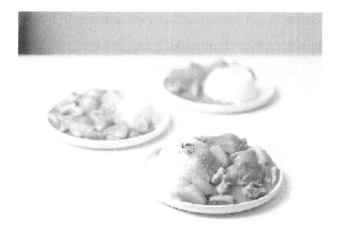

A BLACK BEAN EXTRAVAGANZA

Black bean burgers An excellent substitute for beef burgers, these vegan patties are bursting with taste and protein. Put your favourite burger toppings on top.

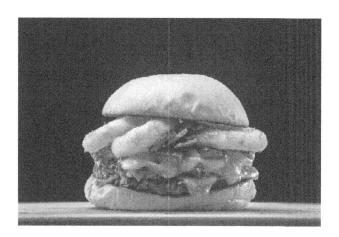

Black Bean Soup: A hearty and flavorful soup with black beans, corn, tomatoes and spices. Perfect for a cozy meal on a chilly day.

Black Bean and Mango Salsa: A refreshing and vibrant salsa with black beans, mango, red onion, and cilantro. Great with tortilla chips or as a topping for grilled fish or tacos.

KIDNEY BEAN FIESTA

Kidney Bean Chili: A hearty and flavorful chili with kidney beans, ground beef (optional), tomatoes, peppers, and spices. A classic comfort food.

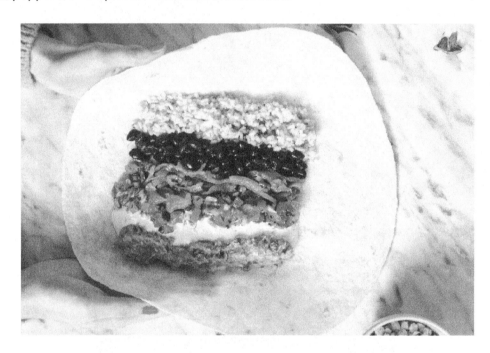

Kidney Bean Salad: A protein-packed salad with kidney beans, quinoa, corn, black olives, and a zesty vinaigrette. Perfect for a healthy and satisfying lunch.

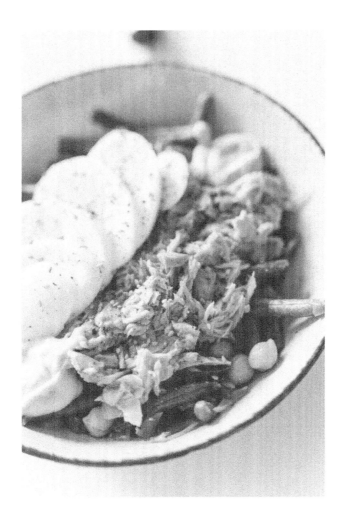

Kidney Bean Burgers: Similar to black bean burgers, kidney bean burgers offer a slightly different flavor and texture. Experiment with different spices and toppings!

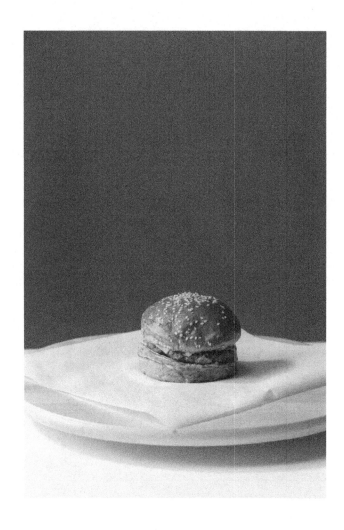

This is just a starting point! The possibilities with beans are endless. So, embrace the culinary adventure, explore new recipes, and discover the delicious and nutritious world of beans!

Bonus Tip: Don't be afraid to experiment with different spices and herbs to personalize your bean dishes. Fresh herbs like cilantro, parsley, and basil add a burst of flavor, while spices like cumin, chili powder, and smoked paprika can create a variety of taste profiles. With their nutritional prowess and culinary versatility, beans are a true gift from the plant kingdom. So, let's give them the starring role they deserve in our kitchens and reap the benefits of a bean-tiful diet!

BERRIES

Berries Nature's Candy in a Culinary Showcase:

Berries are nature's little bursts of sunshine, packed with flavor, vitamins, and antioxidants. They're not just for summer picnics, though! Their versatility shines in a variety of dishes, from breakfast to dessert and even snacks. Get ready to be dazzled by a vibrant and flavorful showcase of berry-based delights!

Breakfast:

Berry-licious Smoothie Bowls: Start your day with a refreshing and energizing smoothie bowl. Blend your favorite yogurt or milk with frozen berries, spinach, and a touch of honey. Top it with fresh berries, granola, and chia seeds for a textural and nutritional powerhouse.

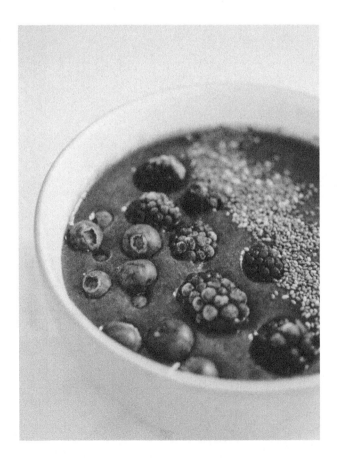

Pancakes with a Berry Burst: Incorporate frozen or fresh berries into your batter instead of using syrup. As the berries boil, their juices will seep out, leaving behind pockets of delectable tartness and sweetness. For a traditional morning treat, garnish with powdered sugar and a dollop of whipped cream.

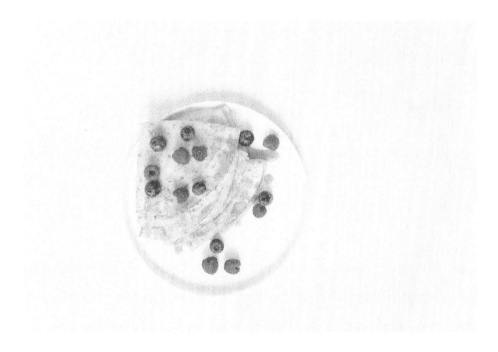

Overnight Oats with Berry Compote: Prepare this quick and easy breakfast the night before. Layer oats, yogurt, milk, chia seeds, and a drizzle of honey in a jar. Top with a homemade berry compote made with simmered berries, lemon zest,vand a touch of sugar. In the morning, you'll have a chilled and flavorful parfait waiting for.

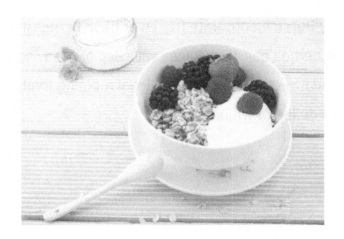

Desserts:

Berry Crumble: This rustic dessert is the perfect way to use up a bounty of summer berries. Toss together berries with a bit of sugar and lemon juice, then top with a streusel made from flour, oats, butter, and brown sugar. Bake until golden brown and bubbly for a warm and comforting treat.

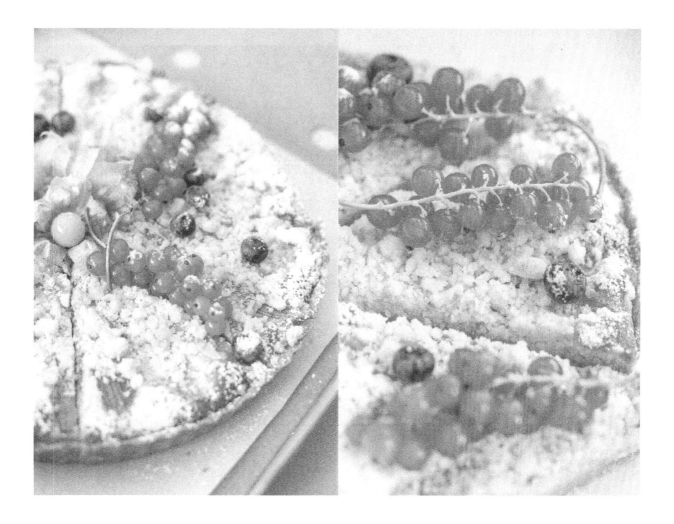

Berry Shortcake: Elevate your berries with fluffy homemade biscuits or storebought pound cake. Whip up some mascarpone cream with vanilla extract and a touch of sweetness. Pile the berries and cream on top of the biscuits, and drizzle with a balsamic reduction for an elegant and impressive dessert.

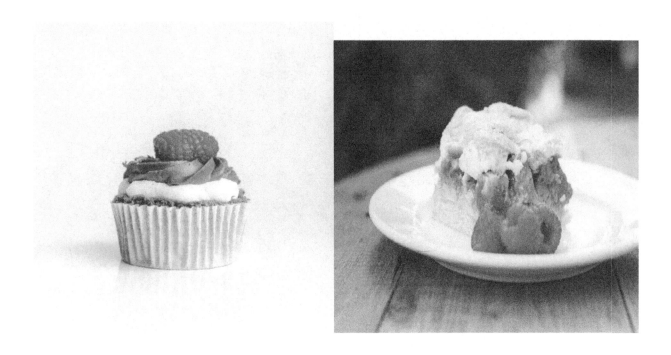

Snacks:

Berry Skewers with Yogurt Dip: Thread fresh berries onto skewers and pair them with a creamy yogurt dip made with Greek yogurt, honey, and vanilla extract. This is a healthy and portable snack that's perfect for on-the-go mornings or afternoon pick-me-ups.

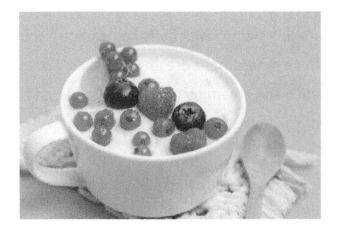

Trail Mix with Nuts and Berries: A homemade trail mix can help you feel more energised. Mix in your favourite berries, nuts, and seeds, as well as dried fruit. You can carry this portable, wholesome snack with you wherever you go.

These are just a handful of suggestions to get you going. There are many ways to use berries in your meals and snacks if you just use a little imagination. So go out, discover the world of berries, and let their vivid tastes and many applications to entice your palate!

Bonus Advice: Don't be scared to try out various berry varieties! Every type has a distinct flavour and texture of its own. To make your own unique fruit meals, try combining blueberries, raspberries, strawberries, blackberries, and other berries. I hope you've been motivated to embrace the culinary enchantment of berries by this thorough exhibition!

GREANS

Now, vegetarian warriors, set down your salad spinner and prepare to unleash the nutritional power of leafy greens! We're going to explore a world of delectable possibilities where greens take centre stage, going beyond the traditional bowl. Get comfortable, as we will be exploring entrées, soups, and smoothies that will transform your connection with these nutrient-dense superfoods.

Principal Courses:

Leafy Green Lasagna: Use sheets of soft kale or collard greens instead of the withered noodles. For a flavorful, nutrient-dense vegetarian lasagna, layer them with ricotta cheese, velvety marinara sauce, and your favourite vegetables.

Stuffed Sweet Potatoes: Stuff those roasted sweet potatoes with a flavorful mixture of crumbled tofu, quinoa, and sautéed kale. Add a generous amount of tahini sauce on top for a nutritious and filling dinner.

Use up leftover kale with this Italian-inspired recipe, Kale & Sausage Frittata. Add chopped kale, eggs, and your preferred vegetables to a pan. Eat a piece for breakfast, lunch, or supper after baking until golden brown.

Soups:

Creamy Spinach & Mushroom Soup: For a filling and healthful soup, blend cooked spinach with earthy mushrooms, creamy cashew butter, and rich vegetable broth. For an additional flavorful layer, add a swirl of pesto on top. Smoky and savoury, Spicy Collard Green Soup will make you feel like you're in the South. For a filling and stimulating dinner, simmer collard greens with black beans, corn, jalapeños, and spices.

Detox Parsley Soup: This soup is light and delicious, perfect for a body cleansing. Mix parsley with ginger, cucumber, celery, and lemon juice for a palate-cleansing and purifying delight.

Smoothies:

The moniker "Green Machine Smoothie" shouldn't scare you! It's astonishing howvsweet and tasty this smoothie is. Blend spinach, almond milk, bananas, and mango to create a nutrient-rich, creamy beverage.

Kale and Berry Cooler: This colourful smoothie will give you an energy boost and plenty of antioxidants. Mix kale, Greek yoghurt, strawberries, blueberries, and honey to make a tasty and hydrating breakfast or snack.

Smoothie with Chocolate Avocado and Spinach: Who says nutritious foods can't be decadent? Smoothie spinach, avocado, banana, cacao powder, and almond milk together to create a rich, creamy, and surprisingly nutritious drink.

Bonus Tip: Keep in mind that adaptability is crucial! Try experimenting with new flavour and texture combinations without fear. Add chopped greens to your favourite pizza crust, use them in stir-fries, or mix them into pancake batter.

There are many options!

So say goodbye to the boring salad and welcome the vibrant world of leafy greens in smoothies, soups, and major dishes. You'll be astonished at how very tasty and fulfilling these meals can be, all while improving your nutritional and physical well-being. Together, with each inventive culinary effort, let's bring greens into the mainstream!

NUTS AND SEEDS

Nuts and Seeds Little Titans of Nutrients and Taste:

Nuts and seeds are nutritious powerhouses, packed full of fibre, protein, and important vitamins and minerals along with healthy fats. Beyond their health advantages, however, they open up a world of gastronomic possibilities by enhancing meals of all types with their distinct flavour profiles, texture, and richness. Today, we're going to look at how to make the most of these little giants, turning them into tantalising toppings, satiating treats, and components that give dips and spreads a whole new dimension.

Add-ons:

Salad Symphony: Never accept blah lettuce! Add a colourful mix of chopped nuts and seeds to your salad. Pumpkin and sunflower seeds lend a nutty richness, while toasted almonds and pecans add a buttery crunch. Pistachios and cashews provide bursts of salty sweetness, while hemp and sesame seeds add a subtle earthiness.

Soup Sensations: A dash of nutty flavour will take your soups from light to hearty. Try adding pine nuts to minestrone, sesame seeds to a spicy Thai lentil soup, or toasted chopped walnuts or pecans to a creamy butternut squash soup.

Oatmeal Adventure: Add a nutty and seedy touch to transform your ordinary oatmeal for breakfast into something amazing. Almonds, walnuts, and pecans provide a delightful crunch, while flaxseeds and chia seeds increase the amount of omega-3 fatty acids. Dates, goji berries, and dried cranberries may provide bursts of tartness and sweetness.

Munchies:

Trail Mix Mastermind: Create your own unique mixes to become a trail mix master. For a pleasing blend of textures, combine seeds like sunflower, chia, and pumpkin with nuts like almonds, cashews, and pistachios. For an added flavour fiesta, add some dried fruit, dark chocolate chips, or shredded coconut.

Nut Butter & Seed Joy: Instead of grabbing store-bought peanut butter, make your own homemade nut or seed butter. Spiralized sunflower seeds, cashews, or roasted almonds are tasty and wholesome substitutes. For a different flavour, try adding a little honey, cinnamon, or cocoa powder.

Roasted Delights: Roasting nuts and seeds makes them tastier and much crunchier. Toss your favourites with curry or chilli powder and a little olive oil,bthen roast till golden brown. For a treat high in protein, try roasted chickpeas.

Dips & Spreads:

Hummus Hero: Give your hummus a makeover with a nutty twist. Add roasted almonds, walnuts, or sunflower seeds to the blender along with chickpeas, tahini, olive oil, and spices. Experiment with different nut combinations for unique flavor profiles.

Spicy Pepita Pesto: Ditch the basil and embrace the pepita (pumpkin seed) in this vibrant pesto. Blend pepitas with cilantro, jalapeños, garlic, lime juice, and olive oil for a spicy and flavorful dip or sauce. Perfect for crudités, sandwiches, or even as a pasta sauce.

Nutty Nut Butter Dip: Blend your favorite nut butter with yogurt, a touch of honey, and spices like cumin or paprika for a creamy and flavorful dip. Serve with apple slices, carrots, or even cucumber slices for a healthy and satisfying snack.

Bonus Tip: Remember, versatility is key! Grind nuts and seeds into flours for gluten-free baking, use them as thickeners in soups and stews, or sprinkle them on yogurt bowls for a satisfying crunch. The possibilities are endless!

So next time you reach for a handful of almonds or sprinkle some seeds on your salad, remember the incredible potential these tiny powerhouses hold. With a little creativity, you can unlock a world of flavor, texture, and nutrition, transforming them from simple snacks to culinary stars. Go nuts and seeds, go!

NUTS AND SEEDS

Herbs and spices are powerful allies in our pursuit of health and wellbeing, not merely culinary partners. These aromatic powerhouses not only give our food layers of flavour, but they also contain a plethora of bioactive substances that fight inflammation, prevent chronic illnesses, and improve general health.

Together with tasting some delectable dishes that highlight these plants' strong flavour and health benefits, let's investigate the science behind these botanical gifts.

Inflammation Warriors: From diabetes and heart disease to cancer and Alzheimer's, chronic inflammation is the cause of many contemporary illnesses. Herbs and spices enter the fray as organic anti-inflammatory warriors. Our cells and tissues are shielded against inflammatory pathways by substances like capsaicin found in chilli peppers, gingerols in ginger, and curcumin found in turmeric.

Heroes of Health: Herbs and spices have many advantages beyond just reducing inflammation. Garlic decreases cholesterol and stimulates the immune system, while cinnamon increases insulin sensitivity and controls blood sugar. Strong antioxidants like rosemary and oregano combine with natural detoxifying properties like parsley and cilantro. Every aromatic companion offers a distinct combination of health-enhancing characteristics.

Tasty Recipes: Let's now use this scientific understanding into enticing recipes:

Golden Turmeric Latte: This cool drink is a powerful source of anti-inflammatory benefits and isn't simply a hipster craze. Mix turmeric powder, ginger, cinnamon,and honey with steaming milk to create a cosy, warm beverage that is also very nutritious.

Mediterranean Salmon with Herbs: Use oregano and rosemary's antiinflammatory properties to enhance grilled salmon. Stuff its guts with garlic, lemon slices, and these strong-tasting herbs for a tasty and nutritious main meal.

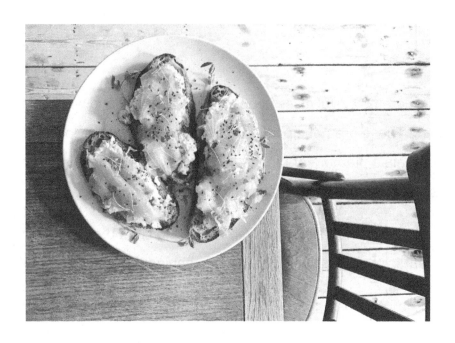

Spiced Lentil Soup: Lentils are protein and fiber champions, while spices like cumin, coriander, and chili peppers add anti-inflammatory benefits and warm depth to this vegetarian staple. A bowl of this hearty soup is a nourishing feast for the body and soul.

Blended Green Goddess Smoothie with Garlic: This antioxidant-rich smoothie will help you start the day with a bright smile. Blend spinach, avocado, pineapple, banana, and a good dose of garlic to make a tasty, detoxifying green smoothie that's not to be missed.

Bonus Advice: Take risks! Combine different herbs and spices to produce unique flavour profiles and gastronomic creations that are health-promoting. Recall that adding even a little amount of these powerful chemicals may have a significant impact on flavour and health.

Accept the power of herbs and spices, then. They're powerful allies in advancing health and wellbeing, not merely taste enhancers. Allow their colourful hues to adorn your dish, their enticing scents to fill your kitchen, and their nourishing qualities to feed your body. Good health and bon appétit!

WHOLE GRAINS

Whole Grains The Natural Superfoods for Filling and Healthy Meals

Put an end to dull and uninteresting! Culinary chameleons, whole grains are plethora of health advantages, flavour, and texture. These nutrient-dense, highfiber jewels provide minerals like iron, magnesium, and B vitamins that support gut health, prolong feelings of fullness, and even decrease cholesterol and the risk of chronic illnesses. So let's put an end to processed grains and explore the scrumptious and healthful possibilities of whole grains like quinoa, oats, and brown rice!

Quinoa Power Bowl: This high-protein power bowl is an ideal platform for experimenting with different recipes. Begin with a bed of light quinoa, then add roasted veggies such as peppers and zucchini, chopped fresh herbs, black beans for extra protein and a squeeze of lime for some flavour. Add some avocado salsa or creamy tahini dressing over top. And voilà! A colourful, filling dinner that stimulates your senses and fills your body up.

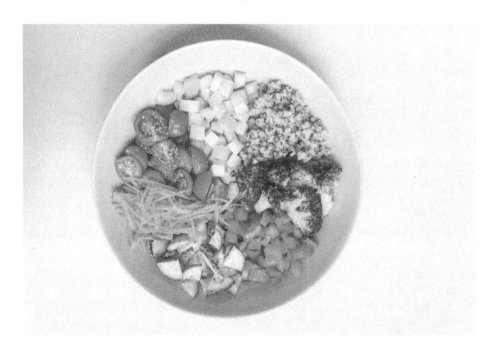

Savory Oatmeal Risotto: Who says oatmeal is just for breakfast? This creamy and comforting dish reimagines oatmeal as a versatile dinner contender. Sauté shallots and garlic in olive oil, then add your favorite broth and simmer until creamy. Stir in cooked oats, Parmesan cheese, and seasonal vegetables like asparagus or mushrooms for a satisfying and flavorful main course.

One-Pot Brown Rice Pilaf: This fuss-free recipe is perfect for busy weeknights. Sauté onions and garlic in a pot, then add spices like cumin, turmeric, and coriander for a warm and fragrant base. Stir in rinsed brown rice and your favorite chopped vegetables like carrots and peas. Pour in vegetable broth and simmer until fluffy and flavorful. This one-pot wonder is a nutritious and hassle-free dinner solution.

CRUCIFEROUS VEGETABLES

The broccoli woods, cauliflower clouds, cabbage fields, and Brussels sprout galaxies of the vegetable world are known as cruciferous vegetables, and they have a hidden weapon in the battle for good health. These nutritious giants, full of vitamins, minerals, fibre, and powerful phytochemicals like glucosinolates (which may be transformed to sulforaphane, a strong cancer-fighting agent), deserve a place of honour in your kitchen that goes beyond the boring limitations of a steamer. Together with our crusaders who are cruciferous, let's throw out the mush and go on an inventive, tasty adventure!

Broccoli:

Past the blossoms: Save those stems! You may spiralize them to make healthy pasta substitutes or roast them with seasonings to make nutrient-dense, crispy fries.

Power of the rainbow: Accept the visual and gustatory delight that is romanesco broccoli, with its fractal beauty and somewhat sweeter flavour. worldwide fusion For a simple side dish with an Asian flair, stir-fry broccoli florets with ginger, garlic, and tamari. Alternatively, blend them into pesto for a distinctive take on pizza or pasta.

Lettuce:

Rice revolution: Using a food processor, pulse florets to make a multipurpose "rice" basis that can be used for sushi, bowls, and stir-fries.

Pizza excellence: For a guilt-free pizza night, roast cauliflower steaks and top with mozzarella, marinara sauce, and your favourite vegetables.

Cheese and cauliflower macaroni: For a traditional vegan comfort food dish, blend cooked florets with cashew cream, nutritional yeast, and seasonings.

Cabbage:

Kimchi kick: A spicy, probiotic-rich condiment made by fermenting shredded cabbage with garlic and spices.

Coleslaw remix: For a bright and energising salad, replace the mayo with shredded cabbage, apples, and walnuts tossed in a tart vinaigrette.

Full and content: To make a filling and savoury main dinner, hollow out the heads of cabbage and stuff them with quinoa, lentils, and veggies.

Brussels Sprouts:

Crispy caramelization: For a savoury and sweet side dish, roast Brussels sprouts cut in half and toss with olive oil and balsamic vinegar.

For a mouthwatering appetiser, toss roasted Brussels sprouts with a maple mustard sauce that combines sweetness and tanginess. Thin slices of dehydrated Brussels sprouts provide a nutritious and very tempting substitute for potato chips.

Extra Advice:

Spice things up: To give your recipes more depth and complexity, try experimenting with herbs and spices like za'atar, cumin, turmeric, and chilli flakes.

Eat uncooked: Savour shredded cabbage in slaw or salads, or cut broccoli stems into sticks and serve them with tahini dip or hummus.

Roast with assurance: Roasting cruciferous veggies intensifies their inherent sweetness and caramelises their edges, imparting a deeper flavour.

Be inventive: Don't be scared to try out new culinary techniques and combinations. There are many options!

Recall that include cruciferous veggies in your diet is about accepting a world of flavour, brilliant colours, and potent health advantages rather than merely following trends. Now get out your chopping board, embrace your inner food activist, and get involved! You are becoming healthier and tastier with every cruciferous invention you make.

SOYBEAN SYMPHONY

Uncovering the Tasty Variety of Soy in Your Everyday Recipe

In the realm of cooking, soy—the lowly bean with a golden heart—or rather, protein—deserves a standing ovation. It is not only a plant-based superfood that is abundant in fibre, protein, and other vital minerals, but it is also very versatile!

Let's break free from the tofu scramble routine and explore the limitless possibilities of soy in your kitchen by immersing ourselves in a soy symphony.

Tofu:

Texture Tango: Tofu may be baked, pressed, silky, scrambled, or any other way you like. Silken tofu may be scrambled for smooth omelettes, or it can be pressed and marinated for firm tofu kebabs that are competitive with any meat

substitute.

Fusion Worldwide: Savour silky tofu pieces in Thai Tom Yum soup, or prepare a spicy Korean stir-fry with crispy tofu cubes.

Sweet Surprise: For a surprisingly filling dessert, bake tofu slices with a sprinkling of cinnamon and a drop of maple syrup.

Tempeh:

Nutty Nirvana: For a substantial, high-protein boost, crumble tempeh into meatballs or vegetarian burgers. Any dish gains depth from its nutty flavour.

Masterpiece of Marinating: Tempeh adores marinades! For a savoury Asian flavour, soak it in a mixture of tamari, ginger, and garlic; alternatively, go smokey with paprika and liquid smoke.

Superstar Salad: If you're wanting something crispy, tempeh bacon bits provide a plant-based substitute. Crumbled tempeh adds structure and protein to salads.

Edame:

Snacking Addiction: Edamame is a versatile and very healthful food that tastes great whether roasted with spices, steamed and dusted with sea salt, or combined into colourful dips.

The Salad Saviour Add shelled edamame to salads to add a burst of texture and extra protein.

Soup Surprise: To add a creamy, high-protein touch to your favourite soups, try adding shelled edamame.

Above and Beyond the Basic Four:

Miso Magic: Soups, stews, and marinades benefit from the umami depth that miso paste, a fermented soybean product, brings. Try a variety of miso types to get a range of flavour characteristics.

Let the doubters begin: A popular Japanese morning meal is natto, which is fermented soybeans with a pungent smell. The stench should not deter you—there are several nutritional advantages!

Tempeh Tempehlah: The options are endless: tempeh hot dogs, tempeh jerky, even tempeh bacon! Accept the adaptability of tempeh by trying these plantbased substitutes for well-known favourites.

Extra Advice:

Add some spice: Spices and herbs have a powerful ability to change soy-based meals. Try out several combinations until you have the ideal flavour profile.

Taste of sauce: For more taste and moisture, drizzle marinades, stir-fry sauces, or salads over your soy creations.

Tofu press to wow: Purchasing a tofu press will assist eliminate extra water from tofu, resulting in firmer tofu with a better texture.

Accept the leftovers: Soy-based meals often improve in flavour the following day! Utilise your creativity while repurposing leftovers to create fresh dishes.

RECIPES FOR EVERY OCCASION

Conquering the kitchen requires not just culinary flair, but also savvy organization. Grouping recipes by meal type and incorporating thematic sections can transform your recipe collection from a chaotic jumble to a well-oiled machine, fueling your day with delicious and inspiring meals.

Breakfast

Quick & Easy: Sheet pan meals with chicken and vegetables, stir-fries, pasta with pesto and tomatoes, salmon with roasted asparagus.

One-Pot Wonders: Slow cooker chili, chicken pot pie, baked salmon with potatoes, creamy tomato pasta.

Seasonal Feasts: Summer grilled steak with grilled vegetables, fall butternut squash soup with roasted chicken, winter beef stew with potatoes and carrots, spring salmon with asparagus and lemon.

Global Flavors: Japanese teriyaki chicken with rice, Indian butter chicken with naan, Moroccan tagine with lamb and vegetables, Italian lasagna.

Desserts & Treats: Homemade ice cream, fruit crumble, chocolate chip cookies, baked apples with caramel sauce.

Snacks:

Quick & Easy: Edamame, apple slices with peanut butter, carrot sticks with hummus, nuts and seeds.

One-Pot Wonders: Yogurt parfait with granola and fruit, hard-boiled eggs, smoothie bowl.

Seasonal Feasts: Fresh fruit and vegetables with dip, roasted pumpkin seeds, airpopped popcorn with cinnamon and honey, homemade trail mix with dried fruits and nuts.

Global Flavors: Edamame with chili flakes, Mexican guacamole with tortilla chips, Indian samosas, Japanese edamame salad.

Desserts & Treats: Dark chocolate squares, frozen yogurt bark, homemade popcorn with spices, yogurt with granola and berries.

BEYOND THE PLATE

Meal planning may make all the difference for busy individuals who are trying to achieve their health goals. Organising ahead of time and being prepared may help you save money, time, and the stress of wondering "what's for dinner?". To ensure success, a little but crucial amount of preparation is necessary before any chopping or grilling occurs. With the knowledge of an experienced dietitian and tips to improve your culinary journey, let's tackle pre-meal prep.

Procurement Skill:

Organise your diet: You may base your grocery list on recipes or a broad theme, such as Mediterranean week. Assess nutritional needs and preferences. Impulsive shopping and food waste may both be decreased with planning.

Recognise the season: Seasonal vegetables are tasty, nutrient-dense, and sometimes less expensive. Check out the farmers market or CSA box in your area for inspiration.

Look over the labels: Avoid foods high in salt, hidden sugars, and unhealthy fats. Choose complete carbs over processed ones and lean protein sources instead.

Bulk up: Acquire necessities like grains, beans, and nuts in bulk to save money and for convenience. Section them off for later use, one at a time.

Recall that frozen food retains nutrients and offers variety. Fruits and vegetables are often flash-frozen at their peak

Shrewd storage:

Store in a cool place: Most fruits and vegetables perform best in the crisper drawer, but leafy greens stay best in sealed containers. Cold and dark storage is ideal for root vegetables.

Welcome sealed containers: Transfer cooked ingredients or bulk-bought items into airtight containers to preserve freshness and prevent rotting.

Management of portions: Portion foods and snacks into different containers in advance to control portion sizes and prevent overindulging. Leading the way, trailing behind: Label and date the things you have saved to prevent waste and to ensure that the older goods are used first.

Blanch and freeze: Vegetables may be blanched prior to freezing, which will inhibit enzyme activity and preserve texture and taste. Excellent for cooking!

Ability to Get Ready:

Over the weekend, prepare large amounts of grains, beans, and proteins. They are perfect for a week's worth of recipes.

Fast-forward until the very last moment: Wash and chop produce over the weekend to use in smoothies, stir fries, and fast salads.

Take a seductive turn: To enjoy with meals throughout the week, make a big batch of your favourite nutritious sauce or dressing.

Hard-boiled utopia A fantastic addition to salads or quick snacks, hard-boiledveggs are a terrific source of protein. Cook some over the weekend for easy access.

Spice up magic: To enhance taste and tenderness, tofu or meats may be marinated in advance. For eventual usage, parts could be frozen.

Additional guidance

For quick and enjoyable preparation, spend money on high-quality cookware and gadgets (such a food processor and sharp knives). Use up any leftovers! Prepare a new lunch or dinner using yesterday night's leftovers.

Put your creativity to use! Do not be afraid to try experimenting with various tastes and components. Instead of being a chore, cooking should be fun. First and foremost, stay grounded. Gradually increase the amount of preliminary work as you feel more comfortable starting small.

Remember, planning, organisation, and thoughtful storage are the keys to a successful meal prep. If you follow these suggestions and methods, you'll be well on your way to being a culinary expert and giving your body nutritious, delectable meals every day of the week. Get ready like a pro and go forward now!

TAMING THE PORTION MONSTER

People having trouble eating is something I see often. Instead than focusing on "what" to eat, focus on "how much." Portion management can be a stressful battlefield, with our own internal signals often shouting for more and the odds of success appearing to be stacked against us due to crowded plates and enticingvcommercials. But do not be alarmed, my dear friend, because I have wonderful news: attentive awareness, rather than stringent limits, is the key to eating healthily.

Let's first get rid of the diet attitude. While stressing about portion sizes and counting calories may temporarily improve one's mood, they eventually damage one's connection with food. Let's concentrate on providing our bodies with nourishment and cultivating a healthy connection with the act of eating instead.

Let's now explore the topic of mindful eating:

1. Pay attention to the murmurs in your body: Think to yourself, "Am I truly hungry, or am I bored, stressed, or craving comfort?" before going for a platter.

Acknowledge emotional eating and look for other healthful methods to satisfy your needs. Take a few deep breaths, find a quiet place to sit, and focus only on your food.

2. Make friends with your plate: Use smaller dinner plates instead of those huge ones. It's an easy approach that uses visual clues to make a lesser piece seem more appetising. Imagine your plate to be split into three sections: one quarter for protein, one quarter for whole grains or starchy vegetables, and one half for non-starchy veggies.

3. Take your time, enjoy the symphony of flavours, and use all of your senses. Chew carefully and set down your fork in between mouthful. Take note of the flavours' gentle dance on your tongue, the textures, and the scents. By taking a deliberate approach, you may stop mindless consuming and learn to actually enjoy your meal.

4. Pay attention to your fullness indicators: Our bodies are quite adept at communicating hunger and fullness signs. Take note of them rather than dismissing them! When you are content but not overstuffed, stop eating. You may always return for more food at a later time if necessary, therefore it's OK to leave some food on your plate.

5. Put an end to your distractions: Mindful eating entails paying attention to what you're eating. Shut down your laptop, put down your phone, and turn off the television. Pay attention to what you're eating and, if any, who you're with.

6. Appreciate diversity: Avoid stigmatising any certain dietary category. Give yourself permission to enjoy every meal in moderation. A varied diet is essential for both balance and enjoyment.

7. Accept the occasional indulgence: There are many parties and sweets in life. If you indulge in an occasional piece of cake or ice cream, don't punish yourself. Savour these moments, enjoy them mindfully, and then return to your mindful eating routine.

Recall that mindful eating is a process rather than a final goal. Even though there will be challenges along the way, every mindful bite is a step in the direction of a happier and better relationship with food. Have faith in your body, pay attention to its signals, and enjoy the pleasure of mindfully and gratefully providing for yourself.

Extra advice:

Meal prep: On hectic days, setting aside portions of your meals and snacks in advance may be very helpful.

Examine food labels: Keep an eye on serving sizes and calorie counts, but try not to obsess over exact amounts. Make use of them as a reference rather than a mandate.

Increase your cooking at home: You now have total control over the components and serving sizes.

Make a movement with your body: Frequent exercise promotes a healthy metabolism and aids with hunger regulation.

I have faith in you. Go out now, and defeat the beast of portions—one mindful bite at a time!

Never forget that I'm here to help you along the road as you adopt mindful eating. Please don't hesitate to get in touch if you need help or have any queries.

CONCLUSION

More than simply a recipe book, "How Not to Age Cookbook" is a colourfulmanual on providing your body with nourishing food that will make you look and feel younger. With this cookbook, you can take control of your health and embrace a thriving future by combining the knowledge of scientific study with delectable flavours.

Highlights of this book that set it apart are as follows:

Scientifically formulated ingredients: Every meal is carefully prepared to include components that have been scientifically shown to promote good ageing. You'll be feeding your cells with every mouthful, from berries high in antioxidants to spices that reduce inflammation.

International inspiration: With a wide variety of tastes and textures to keep your palette happy, the cookbook takes its culinary cues from "Longevity Hotspots" all over the globe.

Easy to make and quite tasty: Healthy cooking is now available to everyone because to the surprisingly simple recipes, which are supported by scientific evidence.

Food alone is not the only thing this book offers; it also provides insights into the science of ageing and useful advice on implementing healthy habits into their daily lives.

Overall, "How Not to Age Cookbook" is a great tool for anybody hoping to age well and have a long, happy life. It serves as evidence of the ability of food to not only fuel our bodies but also provide us the ability to take charge of our health and wellbeing. Open the book, put on your apron, and set off on a tasty trip to a happier, healthier version of yourself.

Made in the USA
Coppell, TX
02 February 2024

28501512R00031